Green Smoothies

Alkaline Green Smoothie Recipes to Detox, Lose Weight, and Feel Energized

By Karen Greenvang

Copyright ©Karen Greenvang

2016

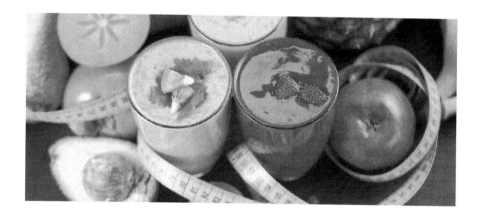

All rights reserved. No part of this publication may be reproduced, stored in a retrieval system, or transmitted, in any form or by any means, electronic, mechanical, photocopying, recording or otherwise, without the prior written permission of the author and the publishers.

The scanning, uploading, and distribution of this book via the Internet, or via any other means, without the permission of the author is illegal and punishable by law. Please purchase only authorized electronic editions, and do not participate in or encourage electronic piracy of copyrighted materials.

All information in this book has been carefully researched and checked for factual accuracy. However, the author and publishers make no warranty, expressed or implied, that the information contained herein is appropriate for every individual, situation or purpose, and assume no responsibility for errors or omission. The reader assumes the risk and full responsibility for all actions, and the author will not be held liable for any loss or damage, whether consequential, incidental, and special or otherwise, that may result from the information presented in this publication.

All cooking is an experiment in a sense, and many people come to the same or similar recipe over time. All recipes in this book have been derived from author's personal experience. Should any bear a close resemblance to those used elsewhere, that is purely coincidental.

The book is not intended to provide medical advice or to take the place of medical advice and treatment from your personal physician. Readers are advised to consult their own doctors or other qualified health professionals regarding the treatment of medical conditions. The author shall not be held liable or responsible for any misunderstanding or misuse of the information contained in this book. The information is not intended to diagnose, treat or cure any disease.

It is important to remember that the author of this book is not a doctor/ medical professional. Only opinions based upon her own personal experiences or research are cited. **THE AUTHOR DOES NOT OFFER MEDICAL ADVICE or prescribe any treatments. For any health or medical issues – you should be talking to your doctor first.**

Table of Contents

Introduction...7

Free Complimentary eBook...12

The Recipes...14

Kale and Cashew Smoothie...15

Cabbage Coconut Chia Smoothie...17

Banana Broccoli Smoothie...19

Apple Carrot Kale Smoothie...21

Spirulina Mango Coconut Smoothie...23

Avocado Blueberry Cherry Smoothie...25

Cocoa Kale Almond Smoothie...26

Orange Coconut Maca Smoothie...27

Barley Grass Lime Smoothie...28

Chia Seed Milk Beet Smoothie...29

Apricot and Cashew Green Smoothie...31

Papaya Cherry Smoothie...33

Watermelon Smoothie...35

Honeydew Smoothie...37

Very Berry Smoothie...39

Pear Smoothie...41

Ginger Smoothie...42

Cocoa Mint Smoothie...44

Chamomile and Kale Smoothie...45

Olive Oil Green Smoothie...47

Lavender Strawberry Smoothie...49

Vanilla Smoothie...51

Cinnamon Smoothie...52

Ashwagandha Coconut Smoothie...54

Grape Smoothie...57

Cucumber Beet Smoothie...58

Celery Green Smoothie...60

Lime Smoothie...62

Arugula Smoothie...65

Ayurvedic Pitta Avocado and Coconut Smoothie...66

Ayurvedic Vatta Berry Almond Smoothie...68

Kapha Apricot and Fig Smoothie...70

Hemp Oil Smoothie...72

Cherry Mint Smoothie...74

Coconut Oil Smoothie...76

Pea and Carrot Smoothie...78

BONUS CHAPTER. Breakfast Jars-Vegan Gluten Free Recipes for Optimal Wellness...79

Conclusion...89

More Vegan Books by Karen...93

Introduction

Green Smoothies have come front and center for a meal choice, snack, or even a dessert. Holistic foods, green leafy vegetables, and proper hydration are hailed in supporting a healthy immune system, excellent energy, and helping ensure longevity. Green smoothies are a part of supporting all three. Best of all green smoothies are delicious and different. They offer an easy alternative to chopping up all the vegetables for a salad. If you drink green smoothies, your energy will increase, your skin will look better, and most of all you feel good. There are so many different food choices to put in green smoothies, and this book uses the plethora of natural healthy foods to make new and interesting green smoothie recipes.

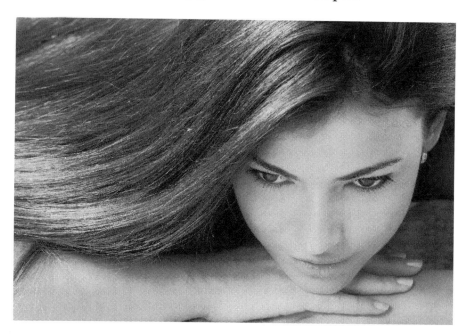

The recipes in this book are full of exciting ingredients. Foods like Spirulina, chia seeds, almond milk, cashew milk, and more. The combinations are endless for making vegan green smoothies, especially with all the great options in the health food stores, and the health food section in regular conventional grocery stores.

The recipes in this book have been especially created for excellent taste and the content of ingredients for your health. None of these green smoothie recipes have dairy or honey in them. The sweetness of these smoothies comes naturally from fruit, and sweet vegetables such as carrots and beets, and other foods that add flavor and texture to the smoothies.

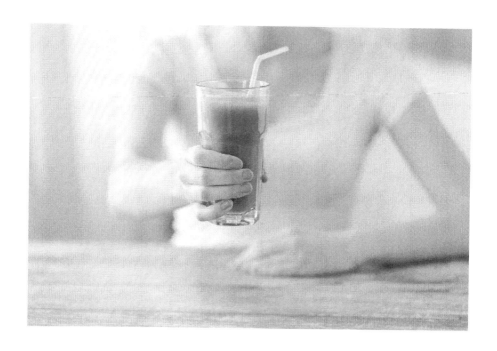

The point of a green smoothie is to get your dose of leafy green vegetables. The smoothies in this book may look one way and taste another. The best thing you can do is make all the smoothies and find the ones that you like the best. There are smoothies in this book that are green and taste more like veggies, and there smoothie recipes where the drink may be green yet taste more like a creamy milk shake. You probably have different tastes at different times. These recipes provide you with these different flavors to satisfy your food cravings in a healthy way.

I congratulate you for choosing to be healthy. Choosing to make a smoothie for a snack or a meal is beneficial to your health and mind. You will be strengthening your bones, muscles, and helping your energy level by making and drinking these smoothies every day, along with healthy exercise you are taking care of yourself. I hope you enjoy the recipes, and now let's take a look at some green smoothie recipes!

This book is not only for vegans or plant-based diet followers. Everyone can benefit from adding more fresh fruits and vegetables into their diet and green smoothies are great for that. If you are not a vegan, but would like to eat more vegan/plant-based, this book will show you how. Everyone is welcome here!

This is going to be an incredibly healthy, holistic journey that will help you explore the green, raw-vegan world. If you would like to improve your health, I suggest you start with a very simple goal- try to have just one green smoothie a day and take it from there. I am not suggesting you should go on a drastic, unrealistic cleanse (all kinds of cleanses and drastic changes to your diet should always be discussed with a medical professional first); all you should focus on is adding. Adding what? More superfood green smoothies. Yummy!

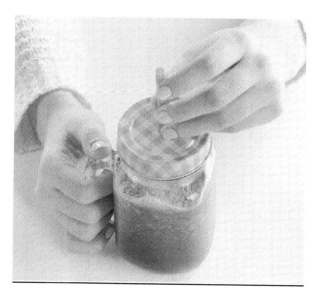
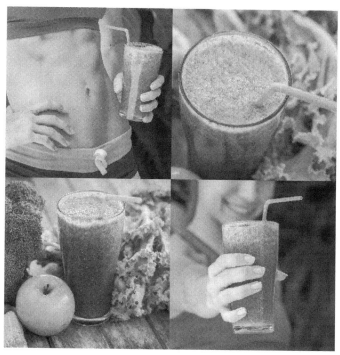

Free Complimentary eBook from Karen

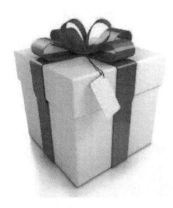

Before we dive into the recipes, I would like to offer you a free, complimentary recipe eBook with delicious vegan superfood smoothies.

Download it now, before you forget.

www.bitly.com/karenfreegift

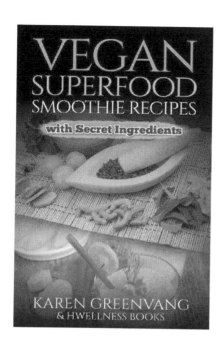

If you have any problems with your download, email me at: karenveganbooks@gmail.com

The Recipes

Recipe Measurements

I love keeping ingredient measurements as simple as possible- this is why I stick to tablespoons, teaspoons and cups.

The cup measurement I use is the American cup measurement. I also use it for dry ingredients. If you are new to it, let me help you:

If you don't have American Cup measures, just use a metric or imperial liquid measuring jug and fill your jug with your ingredient to the corresponding level. Here's how to go about it:

1 American Cup= 250ml= 8 fl.oz

For example:

If a recipe calls for 1 cup of almonds, simply place your almonds into your measuring jug until it reaches the 250 ml/8oz mark.

I know that different countries use different measurements and I wanted to make things simple for you.

Kale and Cashew Smoothie

Serves 1-2

Ingredients

- 3/4 cup of fresh Pineapple
- 1 cup Cold Unsweetened Cashew Milk
- 1 cup of Kale
- 2 drops of Chlorophyll
- ½ cup of crushed ice

Directions

1. Cut the leaves off the top of the pineapple.
2. Cut the spikey skin from the pineapple.
3. Cut the pineapple in four sections by cutting the meat away from the core.
4. Cut up pineapple meat and measure ¾ of a cup of pineapple.
5. Put the crushed ice into the blender and pour in the cold unsweetened cashew milk.
6. Wash the kale.
7. Pull kale leaves away from the stems.
8. Put the kale into the blender along with the chlorophyll. Place the top on the blender and blend on low until everything is mixed.

9. The crushed ice is optional if you would a creamier smoothie. You can taste and add more milk or pineapple if need be. Pour into a glass and garnish with a piece of pineapple on the rim and a straw. Smoothies can be much easier to drink with a straw.

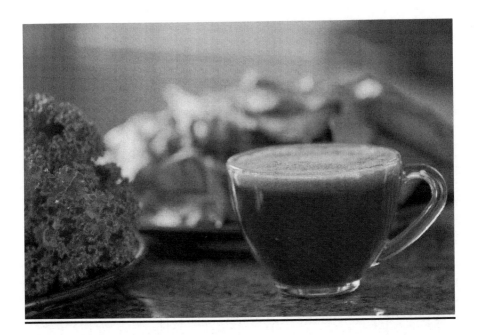

Cabbage Coconut Chia Smoothie

Serves 1-2

Ingredients

- 1/2 cup of cabbage
- 1 cup cold unsweetened coconut milk
- 1 tablespoon of chia seeds
- 1/2 cup of cherries
- 1/2 cup of spinach

Directions

1. Pour the coconut milk into the blender.
2. Cut up the cabbage and put in the blender.
3. Place chia seeds in a coffee grinder and chop to a powder. Brush the powder into the blender.
4. Make sure the cherries do not have pits in them.
5. Place the pit less cherries into the mix.
6. Wash and dry the spinach.
7. Chop up fresh spinach and put in the mix, with the cover on the blender mix on low and them medium.
8. Press puree for a bit and make sure all foods are well blended and copped up.
9. The more you chop up a vegetable before it goes in the blender, the better the mix will be.

10. Taste the blend and see if you like the texture and the flavor. You can gradually add more of any of the ingredients to change the smoothie a little bit. Pour into a glass and enjoy.

Banana Broccoli Smoothie

Serves: 1-2

Ingredients:

- 1 1/2 peeled frozen bananas
- 1 cup almond milk
- ½ cup of cooked broccoli
- ½ cup of kale leaves

Directions

1. Place the peeled bananas in the freezer overnight.
2. In the cut up the bananas and put in blender with the almond milk.
3. Cook broccoli and put in the one half of a cup.
4. You can cook the kale or just put in the raw kale leaves.
5. Wash the kale before use.
6. Make sure to take the leaves off the cores.
7. Throw the cores away.
8. Blend all the ingredients on low until mixed.
9. Then mix ingredient on medium or if there is a puree button.
10. You want everything to reduce down to a smooth consistency.
11. If you need more smooth just add either more almond or a little water is always good as well.

12. Taste the smoothie and add more of any the ingredients if you need to for a slightly different taste.
13. Once you like the smoothie, pour in a glass and serve the smoothie with a straw.

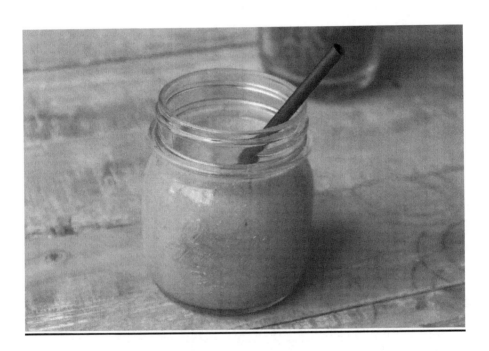

Apple Carrot Kale Smoothie

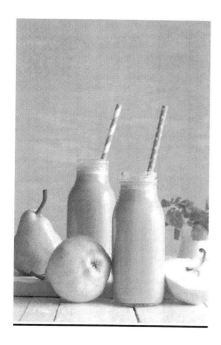

Serves 1-2

Ingredients

- 1 apple of your choice
- ½ cup of carrot juice
- ¾ cup of kale
- 1 teaspoon of fresh ginger

Directions

1. If you have a juicer, juice the apple and ½ cup of carrots and ginger.

2. If you do not have a juicer then buy apple juice that is 100 % apple juice and no sugar added.

The same for the carrot juice.

3. You can buy a container of 100 % carrot juice to do the job.
4. Make sure there is no sugar added.
5. Wash and dry the kale.
6. Pull the leaves away from the cores of the kale.
7. If you do not have a juicer then peel away the outside of the ginger.
8. Add the ginger into mix with all other ingredients.
9. Add the kale to the blender mix and mix on medium.
10. Increase the speed in order to make sure the kale blends up as much as possible.
11. The puree button should help to chop up smaller pieces.

All blenders are different.

12. Once the smoothie is blended, taste and add more of any of the ingredients gradually to change the flavor.
13. Once you have a taste you like pour the smoothie into a nice glass and enjoy with a drinking straw.

Spirulina Mango Coconut Smoothie

Serves 1-2

Ingredients

- 1 teaspoon of Spirulina
- 1 cup of frozen mango
- 1 cup of unsweetened coconut milk
- ½ cup spinach

Directions

1. Cut up the mango the night before.
2. Make sure you peel the skin off of the mango and take out the pit.
3. You want to get the pinkest mango you can for it to be ripe.
4. Put the mango bits in the freezer overnight in a container.
5. In the morning add your frozen mango, cup of unsweetened coconut milk, teaspoon of Spirulina, and spinach to the blender.
6. Put the blender on low to medium and blend until smooth.
7. When smoothie is well blended check the taste, adjust if you need to.

8. When you have the desired taste pour the smoothie in a glass and serve.

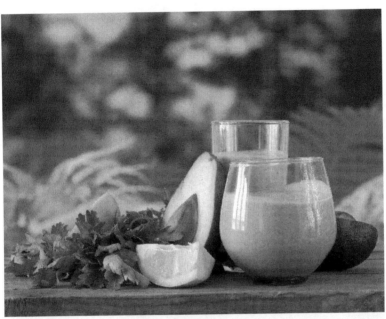

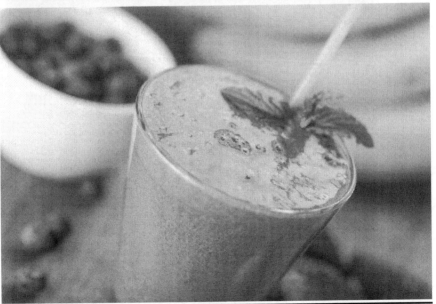

Avocado Blueberry Cherry Smoothie

Serves 1-2

Ingredients

- 1 Avocado soft to the touch
- ¾ cup of fresh then frozen blueberries
- ½ cup of pitted fresh cherries then frozen
- ½ teaspoon lemon
- ½ cup of 100 % no sugar added apple juice

Directions

1. Cut the avocado in half and twist one half avocado gently off of the pit.
2. Spoon the avocado meat into the blender.
3. Pour the apple juice and lemon juice into the blender.
4. Add the cherries and the blueberries to the blender.
5. Blend the mix on low to medium, mixing everything thoroughly.
6. Taste the smoothie and see if you need to add any of the ingredients for taste.
7. When you are ready pour the smoothie into a glass serve with a straw with a straw.

Cocoa Kale Almond Smoothie

Serves 1-2

Ingredients

- 1 tablespoon cocoa powder
- 1 frozen banana
- ½ cup almond milk
- 2 dates
- ½ cup of kale or cabbage

Directions

1. Put the banana in the freezer the night before you will make the smoothie.
2. Peel it first and then put it in a freezer appropriate container.
3. Pour the almond milk into the blender.
4. Pull the leaves of kale away from the stems and cut the kale as small as possible.
5. Put the cut up kale in the blender.
6. Cut the dates in half and take out the pit.
7. Cut the banana in thirds and put in the mix.
8. Blend ingredients together on low to medium.
9. Make sure everything is mixed together, well.
10. Pour into a glass and serve with a straw.

Orange Coconut Maca Smoothie

Serves 1-2

Ingredients

- 1 sweet large orange
- 1 cup of unsweetened coconut milk
- 1 frozen banana
- 1 tablespoon Maca powder

Directions

1. Peel the large orange and cut into four sections.
2. If your orange has seeds in it make sure you that you take the seeds out.
3. You can juice the orange and then throw the remaining seedless pulp into the bender. Just make sure you do not get any seeds in the blender.
4. Pour the coconut milk in the blender along with the cut up frozen banana and Maca powder.
5. Blend everything on low to medium until well blended.
6. Taste a bit to see if you like it and add more of any of the ingredients to change the flavor a bit.
7. When you have the desired taste pour smoothie into a glass and serve with a straw.

Barley Grass Lime Smoothie

Serves 1-2

Ingredients

- 1 to 2 teaspoons of barley grass powder
- ½ cup of frozen raspberries
- ½ cup frozen blueberries
- 1 lime
- ½ cup of apple juice

Directions

1. Pour the apple juice into the blender.
2. Add the frozen raspberries and blueberries to the blender.
3. Squeeze the lime until you have one tablespoon.
4. Put the juice of the lime into the blender.
5. Blend together all the ingredients until they are smooth.
6. Taste the smoothie and see if you like it. If you need to add a little more of the ingredients to suit your taste, do so.
7. When you have the desired taste, cut a ½ inch slice of lime.
8. Cut a slit into the lime and put it on the rim of the glass for garnish.
9. Serve in a glass with a straw.

Chia Milk Beet Smoothie

Serves 1-2

Ingredients

- 2 tablespoons chia seeds
- 2 ¼ cup of water
- ½ teaspoon vanilla
- 1 tablespoon agave syrup
- 3 tablespoons coconut pulp
- ½ cup of beets
- ½ cup collard greens
- 1 peeled pear

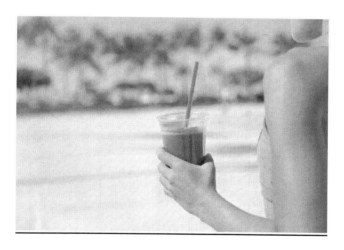

Directions

1. In a coffee grinder or blender make powder out of the chia seeds.
2. The coffee grinder works best.

3. Mix together chia seed powder and the water together in a blender on medium speed. Then add the agave, coconut pulp, and vanilla.
4. Mix everything together in the blender on medium speed.
5. Pour into a glass or bowl and let sit in the refrigerator overnight.
6. In the morning or whenever you are ready to make your smoothie pour 1 cup of chia seed milk and the beets into the blender.
7. Mix the ingredients on low to medium until they are mixed.
8. Then add the collard greens and the peeled pear.
9. Make sure you take the seeds and core out of the pear.
10. Only use the white pear meat.
11. Mix everything on low to medium in the blender.
12. When the ingredients are fully mixed taste the smoothie and if you need to add some more of any of the ingredients go ahead and do so.
13. When you have your desired taste pour the smoothie in a glass and serve with a straw.

Apricot and Cashew Green Smoothie

Serves 1-2

Ingredients

- ¾ cup of fresh, dried or canned apricots
- 1 banana
- ¾ cup of cashew milk
- 2 teaspoons chlorophyll
- 1/4 cup of peas
- 1 date

Directions

1. Put a peeled banana cut in half in the freezer overnight in a container.
2. The next morning cook the peas if they are frozen.
3. If you are using canned peas then you will just put them into the blender.
4. Add the cashew milk, chlorophyll, frozen banana halves, and apricots.
5. Mix in the blender on low to medium until the ingredients are thoroughly mixed.
6. Cut the pit out of the date and put in the blender.

7. Blend the mix on low to medium until everything is smooth and mixed.
8. Taste the smoothie and one or more of the ingredients a little at a time until you get your desired taste.
9. When you like what you taste then pour the smoothie in a glass and serve with a straw.

Papaya Cherry Smoothie

Serves 1-2

Ingredients

- ½ fresh papaya
- ½ cup coconut milk
- 1 teaspoon Spirulina
- ½ cup of cherries
- 1 date

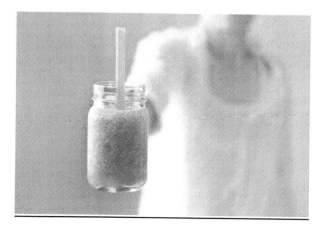

Directions

1. Cut the fresh papaya in half.
2. Take the brown seeds out with a spoon.
3. Cut the green-yellow skin from the outside of the papaya.
4. Cut up the papaya meat from half of the papaya and put it in the blender.

5. Pour the coconut milk into the blender.
6. Spoon the Spirulina in to the mix.
7. Cut up the cherries and take the pits out.
8. Put cherries into the mix.
9. Take the pit out of the date.
10. Put the date meat into the mix.
11. Blend the ingredients in the blender on a low to medium speed.
12. Blend until the mix is blended well.
13. Taste and make sure the smoothie has your desired taste.
14. You can gradually add a little more of one or more of the ingredients to get the taste you desire.
15. When you like the taste of the smoothie serve the smoothie in a nice glass along with a drinking straw.

Watermelon Smoothie

Serves 1-2

Ingredients

- 1 cup of water melon
- ¾ cup of blue berries
- 1 banana
- ½ cup of kale
- 1 teaspoon barley grass
- ½ broccoli

Directions

1. Peel the banana the night before you want to make the smoothie.
2. Put the cut banana in the freezer overnight.
3. Cut the rind off the watermelon and make sure you take the seeds out as well.
4. Cut the water melon into cubes.
5. Put the watermelon in the blender.
6. Add the blueberries and barley grass to the blender.
7. Pull the leaves off the stems of the kale.
8. Add the banana and the kale to the mixture.
9. The broccoli can be put into the blender raw, but it sometimes tastes better if you cook the broccoli first.

10. You can try the smoothies both ways and decide which one you like.
11. Cut the broccoli away from any big stems.
12. But up the broccoli and throw it into boiling water.
13. Let it simmer for no more than five minutes.
14. Cook the broccoli just until it is soft.
15. This allows for the most amount of nutrients to stay in the broccoli.
16. Put the broccoli raw or cooked in the blender with the rest of the ingredients and blend together on low to medium.
17. When the mixture is blended well, serve in a glass with a straw.

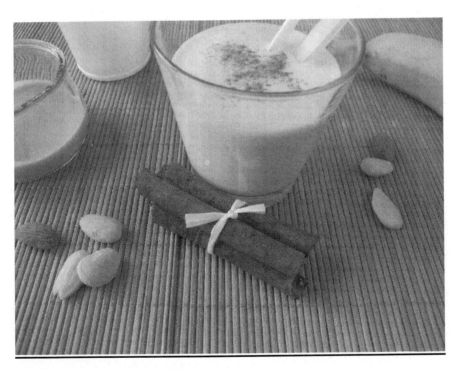

Honeydew Chia Berry Smoothie

Serves 1-2

Ingredients

- 1 cup honeydew melon
- 1 date
- ½ cup of apple juice
- ½ fresh then frozen raspberries
- ½ cup of spinach
- ½ chia seed powder
- 1 teaspoon lemon

Directions

1. Put the fresh raspberries in a freezer appropriate container and place the container in the freezer the night before.
2. When you are ready to make the smoothie take the raspberries out of the freezer.
3. Cut up the honeydew melon and make sure to cut the hard skin from the honeydew melon.
4. Spoon out the seeds before measuring the melon into a cup.
5. Cut the pit out of the date.
6. Pour the ½ cup of apple juice into the blender.
7. Put the date and the honeydew melon into the blender.

8. Then put the frozen raspberries and lemon juice into the blender.
9. Make the chia seed powder in a coffee grinder by grinding the chia seeds.
10. Measure out the spinach leaves and put the spinach and the chia seed powder into the blender.
11. Blend all the ingredients on low to medium.
12. Make sure everything is blended well.
13. Taste to make sure you like.
14. Gradually add more of one or more ingredients if you need to.
15. Pour smoothie in a glass with a straw.

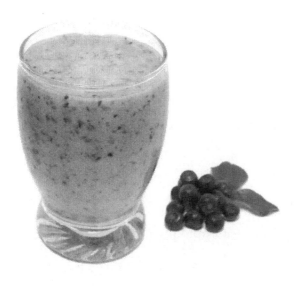

Very Berry Smoothie

Serves 1-2

Ingredients

- 1 cup of fresh then frozen raspberries
- ½ cup of fresh then frozen strawberries
- 2 teaspoons chlorophyll
- 1 cup of cold coconut milk
- ½ cup of kale
- ½ cup of blueberries

Directions

1. Wash the strawberries and raspberries and place them into the freezer overnight.
2. In the morning pour the cold coconut milk into the blender.
3. Take the kale leaves off of the stems.
4. Add the chlorophyll, kale, and blueberries to the blender.
5. Blend all the ingredients together on low to medium speed.
6. Make sure that all ingredients are well blended.
7. Taste and make sure you like the smoothie.
8. If you need to gradually add one or more of the ingredients to the taste.

9. When you are ready pour the smoothie into a glass and serve with a straw.

Pear Smoothie

Server 1-2

Ingredients

- 2 pears
- 1 teaspoon cinnamon
- ½ cup of cashew milk
- ½ cup of apple juice
- ½ cup of melon

Directions

1. Take the two pears wash them and cut the skins off of the outside of the pears.
2. Cut the pears in half and cut the pear meat away from the core of the pear.
3. Put the pear meat into the blender.
4. Measure the ½ teaspoon of cinnamon and put into the blender.
5. Add the cashew milk, apple juice, and melon.
6. Mix all the ingredients together on a low to medium speed.
7. Mix until the ingredients are well blended.
8. Taste your smoothie and gradually add a small amount of ingredients if need.
9. When you like the taste of the smoothie pour the smoothie into a glass with a straw and serve.

Ginger Smoothie

Serves 1-2

Ingredients

- 2 teaspoons ginger
- 2 dates
- ½ cup of kale
- ½ cup of apple juice
- Juice of half of a lemon

Directions

1. Take the ginger and cut the skin from the outside.
2. Take the dates and cut the pit from the center of the dates.
3. Put the ginger and dates into the blender.
4. Pull the kale leaves away from the core.
5. Put the kale in the blender and pour in the apple juice as well.
6. Squeeze the juice of the lemon into a glass and make sure to take out all of the seeds. Then pour the lemon into the blender.
7. Mix all the ingredients in the blender on a low to medium speed.
8. Make sure everything is blended well and copped up as much as possible.
9. Taste and adjust for desired taste if you need to.

10. Pour the smoothie into a glass and serve with a straw.

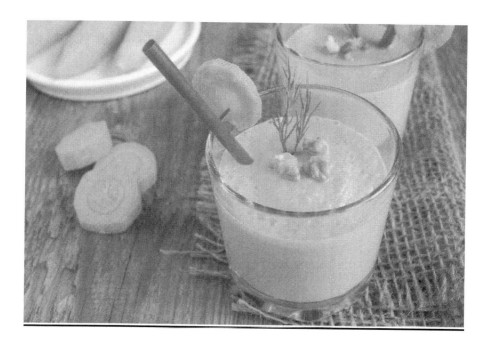

Cocoa Mint Smoothie

Serves 1-2

Ingredients

- ¼ cup of fresh mint
- ½ cup of cold almond milk
- 1 tablespoon of cocoa powder
- 1 banana

Directions

1. Peel the banana and cut it in half.
2. Put the banana in the freezer in a freezer appropriate container the night before making the smoothie.
3. Wash the mint and cut the mint as small as you can.
4. Pour the almond milk in the blender.
5. Put the mint, the tablespoon of cocoa powder, and the frozen banana in the blender. Blend on low to medium until all the ingredients are as small as they can be and everything is blended well.
6. Taste and adjust if you need to.
7. Pour the smoothie into a glass and drink with a straw.

Chamomile Kale Smoothie

Serves 1-2

Ingredients

- 1 cup of chamomile tea
- ½ cup of almond milk
- ½ banana
- ½ cup of kale
- 2 date
- ½ cup of brewer's yeast

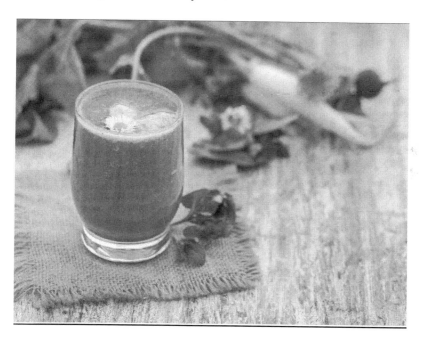

Directions

1. Buy a strong healthy good quality chamomile tea.

2. Make a cup and put two tea bags in so that the chamomile gets a nice and strong flavor. Put the chamomile tea in the refrigerator so it cools before you make the smoothie.
3. You can make the tea the night before.
4. When it is time to make the smoothie pour the almond milk in the blender.
5. Peel the banana and add it to the blend.
6. Pull the kale leaves away from the stems and add ½ cup of kale to the mix.
7. Cut the dates in half and remove the pits.
8. Put the brewer's yeast and dates into the blender.
9. Mix all the ingredients in the blender until they are all well mixed.
10. All the ingredients should be in the smallest form possible.
11. Taste and adjust smoothie by gradually adding one or more ingredients if you need to.
12. When the smoothie is ready pour it into a glass and serve smoothie with a straw.

Olive Oil Green Smoothie

Serves 1-2

Ingredients

- 1 tablespoon olive oil
- ½ cup of apple juice
- ½ cup of broccoli
- ½ cup of artichokes
- ½ cup of kale
- ½ cup of arugula
- 1 pear
- Dash of salt

Directions

1. Cook the broccoli so it is soft.
2. Buy artichokes in a glass container.
3. Add olive oil, apple juice, broccoli, and artichokes to the blender and mix on low to medium.
4. Then pull the kale leaves from the kale stems.
5. Cut the pear in half and peel away the skin.
6. Then cut away the core and stem.
7. Put pear meat and the kale into the blender and mix on low to medium.
8. Put the dash of salt in with the ingredients.

9. Mix all the ingredients until they are all in small pieces and the liquid is smooth to drink. Taste and adjust if you need to. When the smoothie is ready pour the smoothie into a glass with a straw.

Lavender Strawberry Smoothie

Serves 1-2

Ingredients

- 1 teaspoon of culinary lavender
- 2 cups of water
- 2 sprigs of mint
- ½ cucumber
- ½ cup of Strawberries
- 1 teaspoon Spirulina

Directions

1. In a large glass jug add the teaspoon of culinary lavender and the 2 cups of water.
2. Put the two sprigs of mint into the jug.
3. Put in the refrigerator for two hours and take out the sprig of mint.
4. Then keep the lavender mixture in the refrigerator for three more hours.
5. Then strain the lavender from the water.
6. Add lavender water to the blender.
7. Peel the cucumber and measure out ½ cup of cucumber meat and put it in the blender. Cut the green leaves off of the strawberries.
8. Also add the strawberries and Spirulina to the blender.

9. Mix all the ingredients together until smooth and well blended.
10. Taste and adjust if you need to.
11. Serve the smoothie in a glass cold with a straw to drink.

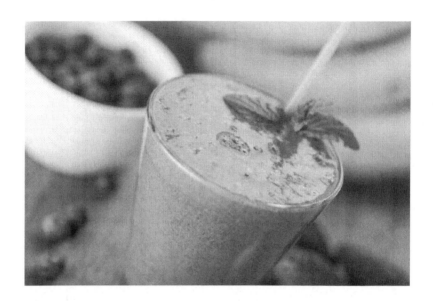

Vanilla Smoothie

Serves 1-2

Ingredients

- 1 natural vanilla bean
- ½ cup of cashew milk
- ½ banana
- 2 tablespoons brewer's yeast
- ½ cup of kale

Directions

1. Take the vanilla bean and press it flat with your fingers.
2. Then take a knife and gently split the vanilla bean open and scoop out the fresh vanilla specs with a spoon.
3. Pour the cashew milk into the blender.
4. Peel the banana and put the banana into the blender.
5. Then put the vanilla and the brewer's yeast in the mix.
6. Also separate the kale leaves from the stems and add the kale to the blender as well. Turn the speed on low and gradually use medium in order to blend all the ingredients together.
7. Blend the mix well so everything is pureed. When smoothie is at desired flavor, pour the smoothie into a glass and serve with a straw.

Cinnamon Smoothie

Serves 1-2

Ingredients

- 2 teaspoons of cinnamon
- ½ cup of almond milk
- 1 apple
- ½ cup of broccoli
- 1 teaspoon barley grass

Directions

1. Cook the broccoli just until it is soft.
2. Pour the almond milk in the blender.
3. Add the ingredients of cinnamon and broccoli along with the barley grass.
4. You can buy fresh cinnamon sticks and grate the cinnamon sticks with a grater until you have enough to fill two teaspoons.
5. Take the peel off of the apple and remove the seed, stem, if it has one, and the core.
6. Put the apple meat into the blender.
7. Turn the blender speed to low and gradually raise to medium.
8. Mix all of the ingredients together until well blended.
9. Taste your smoothie and adjust if you need to by adding a small amount of one or more of the ingredients.

10. When you have your desired flavor, pour the smoothie into a glass and serve with a straw.

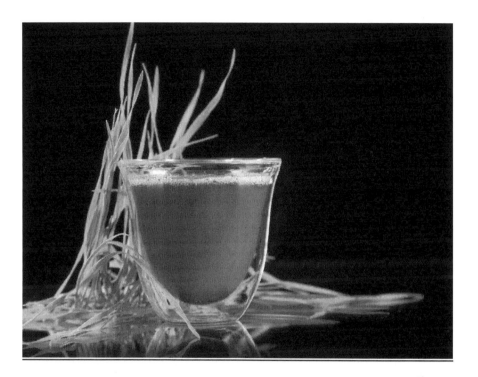

Ashwagandha Coconut Smoothie

Serves 1-2

Ingredients

- 1 teaspoon of Ashwagandha powder
- ½ coconut milk
- 1 frozen banana
- 1 apple
- 3 dates
- ½ cup of blue berries
- ½ teaspoon of lime juice

Directions

1. Warm up the coconut milk in a stainless steel pan on a medium heat.
2. Add the Ashwagandha powder to the warm milk and stir while it is on a low heat.
3. Put the mixture in the refrigerator to cool.
4. You can make the Ashwagandha and coconut mix the night before.
5. Peel the apple and remove the stem and core.
6. Remove the pits from the dates and put the dates in the blender.

7. Add also the lime and apple meat.
8. Mix all the ingredients on a low to medium speed.
9. Mix them well so that all the flavors mix together.
10. Try the smoothie and add a little of one or more ingredients if it needs it.
11. When the smoothie is ready pour the smoothie into a glass with a straw.

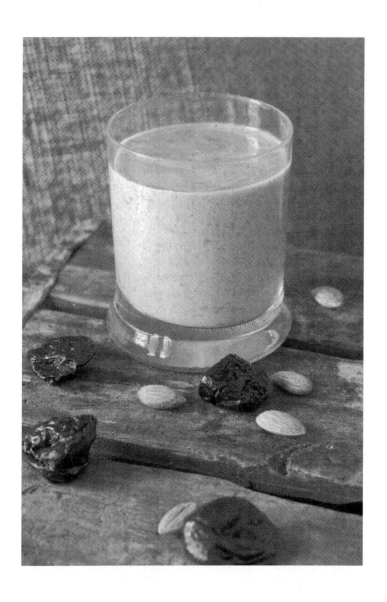

Grape Smoothie

Serves 1-2

Ingredients

- 1 cup of seedless grapes
- 1 pear
- ½ cup of cranberry juice
- ½ cup of broccoli

Directions

1. Put the grapes into the blender.
2. Take the skin off of the pear and take out the core and the stem.
3. Put the pear meat into the blender along with the cranberry juice.
4. Cook the broccoli just until soft, then cool the broccoli in the refrigerator.
5. Put the broccoli in the blender with the other ingredients.
6. Put the speed on low to medium and mix together the ingredients until they are well blended.
7. Try the smoothie and add a small amount of one or more of the ingredients.
8. When the smoothie is ready pour the well-blended mix in a glass and serve with a straw.

Cucumber Beet Smoothie

Serves 1-2

Ingredients

- ¾ cup of cucumber
- ½ cup of beets
- 1/2 cup of hemp milk
- ½ cup arugula
- ½ teaspoon of lime
- Dash of salt

Directions

1. Peel the skin off the outside of the cucumber.
2. Cut up the cucumber, measure and put the cucumber in the blender.
3. Cut up the beets and put the beets in the blender.
4. Pour the hemp milk in the mix.
5. Cut up arugula and put in the blender.
6. Squeeze a lime and put the ½ a teaspoon in the mix.
7. Add the dash of salt.
8. Mix all the ingredients in the blender on low to medium.
9. Blend until all the ingredients are smoother than a puree.

10. Taste and add one or more of the ingredients if you need the change.
11. Once you get the flavor you desire pour the smoothie into a glass and serve with a straw.

Celery Green Smoothie

Serves 1-2

Ingredients

- ½ cup of celery
- ½ cup of broccoli
- ½ cup of carrot juice
- 1/2 cup of unsweetened apple juice
- ¼ teaspoon olive oil
- Dash of salt
- ½ teaspoon apple cider vinegar
- 1 teaspoon of chia seeds

Directions

1. Cut the celery into four sections.
2. Cook the broccoli just until it is soft.
3. Either buy a carrot juice from the refrigerated section in the produce section of the grocery store or juice ½ lbs. of carrots.
4. Pour carrots juice into the mixture.
5. Buy unsweetened not from concentrate apple juice, apple cider is great too.
6. Pour the apple juice into the blender.
7. Add the olive oil, salt, vinegar, and chia seeds.

8. Mix together the ingredients on a low to medium speed until everything well mixed together.
9. Taste your smoothie and if you need to add a little of one or more of the ingredients feel free to do so.
10. Once you get the flavor you want, serve the smoothie in a glass with a straw.

Lime Smoothie

Serves 1-2

Ingredients

- ½ cup of celery
- 2 tablespoons of lime
- 1 tablespoon of lemon
- ½ cup of crushed ice
- 1/2 teaspoon chlorophyll
- ½ cup of kale
- ¼ cup of apple juice

Directions

1. Wash the celery and cut up the stalk to make the ½ a cup.
2. Cut the lime in half and squeeze the juice out to measure.
3. You might have to buy two limes to come up with the two tablespoons.
4. Cut the lemon in half to measure out the one tablespoon.
5. Put the celery, lime juice, and lemon juice into the blender.
6. Pour the crush ice into the blender.

7. Pull the leaves of kale off of the kale stems and put the kale into the blender as well. Pour the apple juice into the mix.
8. Mix all of the ingredients in the blender on a low to medium speed until everything is well blended.
9. Taste the smoothie and add a little of one or more ingredients if you think it needs it. Once you like the taste, pour in a glass and serve with a straw.

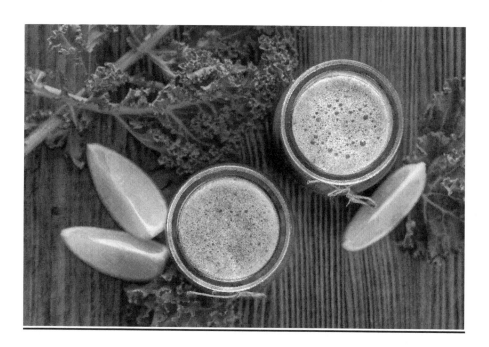

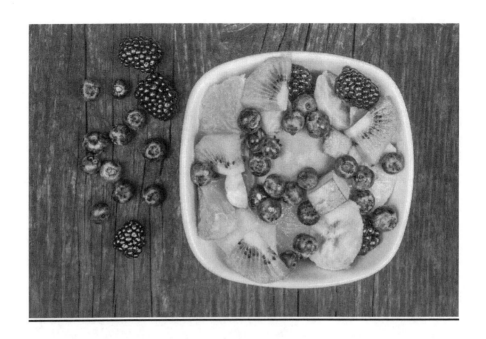

Arugula Smoothie

Serves 1-2

Ingredients

- ½ cup of arugula
- ½ cup of kale
- ½ cup of peaches
- ½ cup of almond milk
- ¼ cup of crushed ice
- 1 date

Directions

1. Wash the arugula and cut it up to measure.
2. Pull the leaves of the kale away from any stems and measure.
3. Cut a peach in half and take out the pit.
4. Take the date and cut the pit out.
5. Pour the ½ cup of almond milk into the blender.
6. Put the arugula, kale and peaches into the blender.
7. Add the crushed ice and date to the blender.
8. Mix all the ingredients on a low to medium speed.
9. Mix the ingredients well until they are pureed and the ingredients are smooth.
10. Pour a serving into a glass and serve with a straw.

Ayurvedic Pitta Avocado and Coconut Smoothie (Relaxing)

Serves 1-2

Ingredients

- ½ cup of avocado
- ½ cup of coconut
- ½ cup of almond milk
- ½ teaspoon of vanilla

Directions

Ayurvedic Pitta is warm to hot and oily in nature so to keep a happy Pitta stomach and system you want foods that are cool and on "the dry side" (in other words; foods that help you cool down your mind, body and temper).

The ingredients in the Pitta Smoothie are researched and approved for the pitta system. Take the avocado and cut the avocado in half and take out the pit.

1. Peel the skin from the outside of the avocado.
2. Put the avocado in the blender.
3. Either buy coconut in a package that has no added ingredients like sugar or sulfur dioxide.
4. If you cannot find dry coconut, you can usually find some in the freezer section.

5. You can also buy a fresh coconut and crack it open with a hammer and screwdriver.
6. Be very careful of course.
7. Poke a hole with the screwdriver and pour out the coconut water in a glass.
8. Strain the water with a strainer.
9. Set the coconut water aside for another smoothie or if you if you need more liquid for this smoothie you can use the coconut water.
10. Place the screwdriver on the side and tap the screwdriver with the hammer until the coconut cracks.
11. When you get a little bit of shell off you, you can then use a butter knife to help get the shell off.
12. Cut the brown skin off of the coconut meat.
13. Cut up enough coconut to measure.
14. Put the almond milk in the blender.
15. Take the vanilla bean and flatten it with your fingers.
16. Then take a knife and cut the vanilla bean longwise.
17. Scoop out the vanilla with a spoon to measure.
18. Mix all the ingredients in the blender on low and then mix on medium.
19. Make sure all the ingredients are thoroughly mixed.
20. When everything is mixed well test a little to see if it tastes good.
21. You can then add more of the ingredients to your liking and texture.

22. When you get the smoothie how you like it, then serve in a glass with a straw.

Ayurvedic Vata Berry Almond Smoothie (Balance, Focus & Relaxation)

Serves 1-2

Ingredients

- ½ cup of blueberries
- ¼ cup of raspberries
- 2 dates
- ¼ cup of watercress
- ½ cup of almond milk

Directions

In Ayurveda, Vata types are known for being cool, dry, and rough and they need foods that are oily, warm, and moist. The foods in this Vata smoothie are tested and approved for the Vata system. They help restore energy and balance- for the mind and body. They help vata's focus better without getting overstimulated.

1. Put both the blueberries and raspberries in the freezer the night before you want to make the smoothie.
2. Make sure you put the berries in a freezer safe container.
3. Pour the almond milk in the blender.
4. Cut the pit out of the dates.
5. Put the dates in the blender.
6. Wash the watercress and measure and put the watercress in the blender.
7. Put both the blueberries and the raspberries in the blender.
8. Mix all the ingredients together in the blender on a low to medium speed.
9. Mix them well and then taste a little of the smoothie.
10. If you want the smoothie thicker add more berries and if you want it thinner add more milk.
11. When you have the desired consistency and taste pout in a glass and serve with a straw.

Kapha Apricot Fig Smoothie

Serves 1-2

Ingredients

- ½ cup of fresh apricots
- 1/4 cup of figs
- ½ cup of fresh vanilla dairy-free vegan yogurt
- ½ cup of cabbage
- ¼ cup of cranberry juice

Directions

In Ayurveda, Kapha is consistent with cool, heavy, and oily so Kapha needs foods that are warm and dry for a nice balancing effect to get more energy for life.

1. Measure out the apricots and put in the blender.
2. Pour the cranberry juice in the blender.
3. Cut up and measure the figs.
4. Add the figs and the vanilla yogurt to the blender.
5. Cut up the cabbage and measure.
6. Put cabbage into the blender as well.
7. Put the cover on the blender and mix on low to medium speed.
8. When the ingredients are well mixed together then taste a little bit and see if you like the consistency and taste.

9. You can thicken with more yogurt or cabbage and thin out with more juice.
10. Once you like the flavor, serve in a glass with a straw.

Hemp Oil Smoothie

Serves 1-2

Ingredients

- 1 tablespoon of hemp oil
- ½ cup of almond milk
- ½ cup of apricots
- ½ cup of carrot juice
- ¼ cup of peaches

Directions

1. Buy carrot juice in the store or if you have a juicer juice ½ lbs. of carrots.
2. Pour the carrot juice in the blender.
3. Also pour the almond milk in the blender along with the hemp oil.
4. Cut up a peach and take the pit out.
5. Also cut up the apricot and take the pit out. Put both fruits into the blender.
6. Blend all the ingredients on a low to medium speed until they are well blended.
7. Taste the smoothie and add one or more of the ingredients if you think it needs it.

8. Once the smoothie tastes the way you want, pour the smoothie into a glass and serve with a drinking straw.

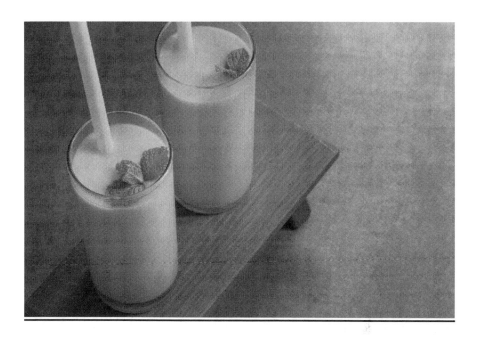

Cherry Mint Smoothie

Serves 1-2

Ingredients

- 3/4 cup of cherries
- 1 teaspoon of mint
- 1/2 cup of almond milk
- ½ cup of kale
- 1/2 teaspoon of fresh vanilla

Directions

1. Wash and cut the cherries.
2. Take the pits out of the cherries.
3. Put cherries into the blender.
4. Pour the almond milk into the blender.
5. Wash the mint and put the two sprigs in the blender.
6. Separate the leaves of kale from the stems.
7. Put the kale into the blender.
8. Press the vanilla bean with your hand and then cut longwise with a knife.
9. With a spoon, scoop out the desired amount of vanilla and put into the blender.
10. Blend all the ingredients together until smooth.

11. Taste your smoothie and if it needs a small amount of one or more of the ingredients then add.
12. When the smoothie tastes to your liking then pour into a glass and serve with a straw.

Coconut Oil Smoothie

Serves 1-2

Ingredients

- 1 tablespoon coconut oil
- ½ cup of cashew milk
- 1 frozen banana
- ½ cup of grapes
- 2 tablespoons Flax seeds

Directions

1. Peel the banana and cut it in half.
2. Put the cut banana in a freezer safe container and freeze overnight.
3. When you are ready to make the smoothie pour the cashew milk in the blender.
4. Put the flax seed in the coffee grinder and make a powder of the flax seeds.
5. Put the frozen banana, grapes, coconut oil, and flax seed powder in the blender.
6. Blend all the ingredients on a low to medium speed.
7. Mix the ingredients until they are smooth.
8. Taste the smoothie and if needs a little extra of one of the ingredients add to the smoothie and remix.

9. When you are happy with the flavor and texture of the smoothie, pour the smoothie in a glass and serve with a straw.

Pea and Carrot Smoothie

Serves 1-2

Ingredients

- ½ cup of peas
- 1 pear
- 1 apple
- ½ cup of carrot juice

Directions

1. Cook the peas until they are soft.
2. Cool the peas in the refrigerator.
3. Wash the pear and cut it in half.
4. Cut away the stem and the core until you are only left with pear meat.
5. Cut up the pear and put the pear meat into the blender.
6. Cut up the apple and take the core and seeds out.
7. Put apple into the blender.
8. Pour the carrot juice into the blender.
9. Mix all the ingredients together until they are smooth.
10. Taste the mixture and if you need to add a little bit of one or more of the ingredients, then go for it.
11. Once you have your desired taste then pour the smoothie into a glass and serve with a straw.

BONUS CHAPTER

Breakfast Jars: Bonus Vegan Gluten Free Recipes for Optimal Wellness

The concept of a pre-made breakfast in a jar is incredibly versatile and time-saving, as it is something that you can prepare the night before and refrigerate until morning. Because the breakfast jar recipes that follow are made in a mason jar and are a gluten-free alternative based on the overnight oats concept, they are a perfect on-the-run breakfast option. The use of Chia seeds instead of oats provides a healthy dose of omega-3's and the added fruits bring in healthy carbohydrates, vitamins and minerals. Each jar is a single serving, so you would need to make one jar per person.

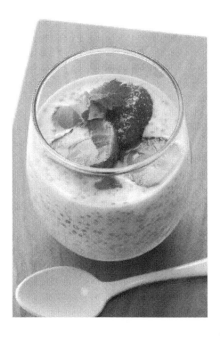

Carrot "Cake" Chia Seed Breakfast Jar

Carrots are a great source of vitamin A, are high in fiber, and a small amount of healthy carbohydrate. The golden sultanas not only add a hint of sweetness, but also are high in vitamin C. The coconut milk and pecan nuts provide a further dose of healthy fats and the ground ginger and cinnamon have anti-inflammatory and immune-boosting properties.

Serves One

Ingredients:

- 2 Tablespoons (30ml) Chia Seeds
- ¼ Cup (60ml) Coconut Milk
- 1 Tablespoon (15ml) Golden Sultanas
- 2 Teaspoons (10ml) Grated Carrot
- 1 Tablespoon (15ml) Raw pecan nuts, chopped
- ¼ Teaspoon (1.25ml) Ground Cinnamon
- ¼ Teaspoon (1.25ml) Baking spice mix
- ¼ Teaspoon (1.25ml) Ground Ginger
- ¼ Teaspoon (1.25ml) Vanilla Essence

Instructions:

1. In a medium-sized Mason jar, mix the Chia seeds, grated carrot, sultanas, ground cinnamon, baking spice mix, ground ginger, and pecan nuts.

2. In a small milk jug, mix the coconut milk with the vanilla essence and pour over the other ingredients that are already in the Mason jar.

3. Mix all ingredients well, making sure that everything is combined and place the lid tightly on the jar.

4. Refrigerate overnight.

5. The idea is to eat this breakfast out of the jar, and it can be served with ¼ cup (60ml) vegan yoghurt (like for example coconut yoghurt).

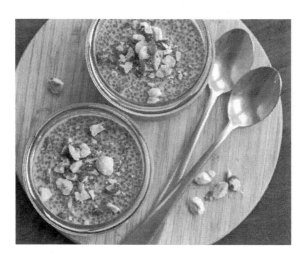

Almond and Banana Chia Seed Breakfast Jar

Bananas are a wonderful source of healthy carbohydrate and their high potassium content makes them an incredibly good source of pre and post workout energy. The almonds are high in healthy fats and protein. The raisins add a little extra sweetness and are a good source of energy and iron.

Serves One

Ingredients:

- 2 Tablespoons (30ml) Chia Seeds
- ¼ Cup (60ml) Almond Milk
- 1 Tablespoon (15ml) Raisins
- 1 small Banana, mashed
- 1 Tablespoon (15ml) Raw almonds, chopped (you can also used raw almond flakes)
- ¼ Teaspoon (1.25ml) Ground Cinnamon
- ¼ Teaspoon (1.25ml) Vanilla Essence

Instructions:

1. In a medium-sized Mason jar, mix the Chia seeds, raisins, mashed banana, ground cinnamon and almonds.

2. In a small milk jug, mix the almond milk with the vanilla essence and pour over the other ingredients that are already in the Mason jar.

3. Mix all ingredients well, making sure that everything is combined and place the lid tightly on the jar.

4. Refrigerate overnight.

5. The idea is to eat this breakfast out of the jar, and it can be served with ¼ cup (60ml) vegan yoghurt of your choice.

Apple Cinnamon Chia Seed Breakfast Jar

Apples are a great source of vitamin C, and their high pectin content makes them incredibly filling and satisfying, making this a fruit a great breakfast addition since it will keep you going all morning. The almond milk in this variation provides a healthy dose of calcium and protein, and by serving it with natural peanut butter you are getting a little extra protein and healthy fats.

Serves One

Ingredients:

- 2 Tablespoons (30ml) Chia Seeds
- ¼ Cup (60ml) Almond Milk
- 1 Tablespoon (15ml) Raisins
- 1 Tablespoon (15ml) Grated Apple
- ¼ Teaspoon (1.25ml) Ground Cinnamon
- ¼ Teaspoon (1.25ml) Baking Spice mix
- ¼ Teaspoon (1.25ml) Vanilla Essence
- 1 Teaspoon (5ml) Natural peanut butter (for serving)

Instructions:

1. In a medium-sized Mason jar, mix the Chia seeds, raisins, grated apple, ground cinnamon and baking spice mix.

2. In a small milk jug, mix the almond milk with the vanilla essence and pour over the other ingredients that are already in the Mason jar.

3. Mix all ingredients well, making sure that everything is combined and place the lid tightly on the jar.

4. Refrigerate overnight.

5. Top with the natural peanut butter before serving

6. The idea is to eat this breakfast out of the jar, and it can be served with ¼ cup (60ml) dairy-free vegan yoghurt of your choice.

Chocolate Berry Delight Chia Seed Breakfast Jar

Strawberries are rich in anti-oxidants and high in vitamin C. Raw cocoa is a super food that is also very high in antioxidants and known for its blood pressure reducing properties. Goji berries that are found in the dried berry mix are also considered a super food, and it is well known that Chia seeds carry the super food label, therefore this breakfast jar is a complete super food guaranteed to start your day in a super way.

Serves One

Ingredients:

- 2 Tablespoons (30ml) Chia Seeds
- ¼ Cup (60ml) Coconut Milk (can be also almond milk, chia seed milk, cashew milk etc.)
- 1 Tablespoon (15ml) Dried Berry mix
- 1 Tablespoon (15ml) Fresh Strawberries, finely chopped
- ¼ Teaspoon (1.25ml) Ground Cinnamon
- 1 Teaspoon (5ml) Raw Cocoa Powder
- ¼ Teaspoon (1.25ml) Vanilla Essence

Instructions:

1. In a medium-sized Mason jar, mix the Chia seeds, dried berry mix, chopped strawberries, ground cinnamon and raw cocoa powder.

2. In a small milk jug, mix the coconut milk with the vanilla essence and pour over the other ingredients that are already in the Mason jar.

3. Mix all ingredients well, making sure that everything is combined and place the lid tightly on the jar.

4. Refrigerate overnight.

5. The idea is to eat this breakfast out of the jar, and it can be served with ¼ cup (60ml) dairy-free vegan friendly yoghurt of your choice.

Don't forget to download your free complimentary eBook.

It's waiting for you at:

http://www.bitly.com/karenfreegift

Download it now, before you forget.

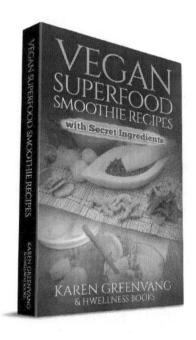

If you have any problems with your download, email me at: karenveganbooks@gmail.com

Conclusion

Making green smoothies is fun and exciting. It also makes a meal that is nutritious, easy to prepare, drink, and clean-up. We all need to save time these days. Making smoothies is also a very quick way to maintain and improve a healthy body. There are so many different combinations to try, you are bound to find three, four, or more you like and want to stick with for a long time. It is important to understand a few things when buying the ingredients for the smoothie. Should you buy organic or conventional fruits and vegetables? If you can afford to buy all organic food, it is in your best interest to do so. If you can afford to buy just some organic foods then buy the one that have the thinnest skin. A food like a banana has a thick skin that can keep out some harmful chemicals. So bananas you will be okay buying conventional.

Frozen over fresh food? It is a good idea to buy fresh foods. Food is always better fresh. The reason to put the food in the freezer for smoothie purposes is to get the smoothie cold. Adding ice to a smoothie can easily make it watery. Putting the food in the freezer before it goes in the blender makes the smoothie cold. There is generally nothing bad about frozen food, as long as it has not been in the freezer too long. Frozen food is a great way to protect food from spoiling.

You might want to know about canned food. Try to eat mostly fresh vegetables and fruits, but if you have to use canned food occasionally, it is fine. Sometimes you may have to use canned because of a seasonal fruit, or it just may be the only way to get a particular item for the smoothie.

It is possible that you may not like a smoothie at first. There is no hard rule about how a smoothie should be made so you can add or subtract any of the ingredients if you don't necessarily like something. Also adding to make your smoothie stronger is a supported situation, because everyone's taste buds are different.

The foods that make up these smoothies are healthy. Not everything good for you tastes good so sometimes you need to hide the flavor with another better flavor. This way you still get the benefits of the food you don't necessarily like, yet you do not have to taste it. You can always add but never take away so add a small amount of the ingredients after you have added the proper measurements.

I congratulate you for making a leap towards a healthy body. You will find that you may get sharper and even faster when you have been drinking these smoothies for about six months.

You will start seeing a difference in your body and mind right away. Remember you can eat other things during the day as well. The smoothie is a great lighter meal or a quick energizing snack (for example before a workout) when the other meals you have can be a bit larger. Smoothies are light and easy meals that pack a world of nutrition in them. I hope you have enjoyed this smoothie book, and that some, if not all of the recipes are good for you. Thank you again for reading!

Karen

PS. If you enjoyed my book, it would be greatly appreciated if you left a review so others can receive the same benefits you have. Your review can help other people take this important step to take care of their health and inspire them to start a new chapter in their lives.

At the same time, <u>you can help me serve you and all my other readers</u> even more through my next vegan-friendly, holistic health recipe books that I am committed to writing.

I'd be thrilled to hear from you. I would love to know your favorite recipe(s).

Don't be shy, post a comment on Amazon!

→ Questions about this book? Email me at: karenveganbooks@gmail.com

Thank You for your time,

Love & Light,

Until next time-

Karen Vegan Greenvang

More Vegan Books by Karen

Available in kindle and paperback in all Amazon stores

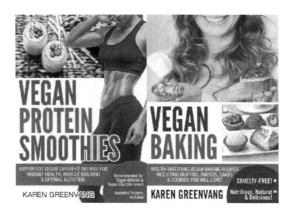

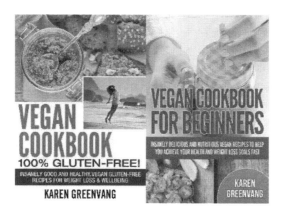

You will find them in your local Amazon store

Made in the USA
Lexington, KY
23 May 2018